Type Two Diabetes

Facts, Diagnosis, Symptoms, Treatment, Causes,
Effects, Prognosis, Research,
History, Myths, and More!

By Frederick Earlstein

Foreword

Diabetes Mellitus is one of the top diseases that dates back to ancient times – at the time of the early Egyptians. Unfortunately, this disorder is one of the most common types of conditions that still exist today. Chances are if you are reading this book, you or any of your loved ones may have been diagnosed with a more specific kind of condition which is Type II diabetes. According to recent statistics, every year there are about 1.4 million people in the U.S. alone who are being diagnosed with diabetes for the first time; people who have Type II diabetes in United States accounts for about 95% out of the 25.8 million cases recorded. Unfortunately lots of people (about 8.1 million) are not receiving proper treatment due to many issues such as lack of awareness and knowledge about the disorder, financial incapacity, or social stigma.

Fortunately, Diabetes, specifically Type II Diabetes is highly treatable and can even be prevented. If you or any of your friends and family is suffering from such illness, it is better gain some knowledge about this condition, so that you'll know how to combat it, and also be able to help others who are suffering from it. This book will provide you with a wealth of information about Type II Diabetes; what it is, its effects, its treatment, and how to deal with it.

Table of Contents

Introduction

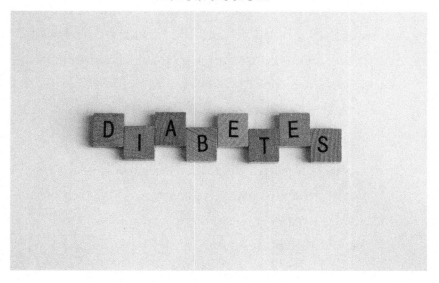

There are about 1.4 million new cases of diabetes in United States annually; and according to researchers the numbers are actually increasing every year. As a matter of fact, 9% of the world's population had diabetes just a few years back according to the estimation of the World Health Organization (WHO). In 2015, an estimated 400 million people worldwide were diagnosed with the disease.

But that's not a surprise anymore to some people, because diabetes has been recognized as one of the deadliest diseases known to human existence. However, what a lot of people don't know is that Type II diabetes accounts for 90% out of the 400 million people diagnosed worldwide.

That statistic only means one thing – many people are diagnosed with Type II diabetes more than Type 1 diabetes both in the U.S. and around the world. According to WHO, Type II diabetes causes about 5 million deaths per year and by 2030 that number is expected to double or triple ranking it as the 7th major cause of death worldwide.

Type II diabetes is one of the root causes that promotes complications which eventually leads to cardiovascular diseases, hypertension, hypoglycemia, kidney failure, liver, pancreatic and gastric conditions, stroke, blindness, dementia, and Alzheimer's diseases just to name a few.

Here's another surprise, Type II diabetes is becoming increasingly common among young people. Although the condition is still more prevalent with seniors (65 years and above), many young people (around 20 years and up) are now being diagnosed with this specific disease and also contributing to that huge percentage every year. Type II diabetes is also common in middle – income or developing countries particularly in Asia where urbanization are rapidly changing lifestyle and food choices.

If you want to know more about this condition, then you've chosen the right book! This book contains some of the basic information regarding diabetes (particularly Type II diabetes): its history, the myths surrounding it, its different types (yes there's more to Type II than you think!), the different symptoms, treatments, diagnosis, and prognosis. We will also look at some of the alternative or complementary treatments available, as well as some unconventional recommendations you can try.

Knowledge is power! What are you waiting for? Turn the page now, so you'll know how to combat this disease inside out!

Glossary

Acesulfame-k: An artificial sweetener used in place of sugar; it contains no carbohydrates or sugar; therefore, it has no effect on blood sugar levels. This sweetener is often used in conjunction with other artificial sweeteners in processed low-calorie foods.

Acetone: A chemical formed in the blood when the body breaks down fat instead of sugar for energy; if acetone forms, it usually means the cells are starved. Commonly, the body's production of acetone is known as "ketosis." It occurs when there is an absolute or relative deficiency in insulin so sugars cannot get into cells for energy. The body then tries to use other energy sources like proteins from muscle and fat from fat cells. Acetone passes through the body into the urine.

Acidosis: Too much acid in the body, usually from the production of ketones like acetone, when cells are starved; for a person with diabetes, the most common type of acidosis is called "ketoacidosis."

Acute: Abrupt onset that is usually severe; happens for a limited period of time.

Adrenal glands: Two endocrine glands that sit on top of the kidneys and make and release stress hormones, such as epinephrine (adrenaline), which stimulates carbohydrate metabolism; norepinephrine, which raises heart rate and blood pressure; and corticosteroid hormones, which control how the body utilizes fat, protein, carbohydrates, and minerals, and helps reduce inflammation.

Adult-onset diabetes: A term for type II diabetes that is no longer used, because this type of diabetes is now commonly seen in children; "non-insulin dependent diabetes" is also considered an incorrect phrase in describing type II diabetes, because patients with this type of diabetes may at some point require insulin.

Advantame: An FDA-approved sugar substitute similar to Aspartame; it can be used as both a tabletop sweetener and as an ingredient in cooking. Advantame can also be used in baked goods, soft drinks and other non-alcoholic beverages, chewing gum, candies, frostings, frozen desserts, gelatins and puddings, jams and jellies, processed fruits and fruit juices, toppings and syrups.

Adverse effect: Harmful effect.

Albuminuria: When kidneys become damaged, they start to leak protein in the urine. Albumin is a small, abundant protein in the blood that passes through the kidney filter into the urine easier than other proteins.

Alpha cell: A type of cell in an area of the pancreas called the islets of Langerhans; alpha cells make and release a hormone called "glucagon." Glucagon functions in direct opposition to insulin -- it increases the amount of glucose in the blood by releasing stored sugar from the liver.

Anomaly: Birth defects; deviation from the norm or average.

Antibodies: Proteins that the body produces to protect itself from foreign substances, such as bacteria or viruses.

Antidiabetic agent: A substance that helps people with diabetes control the level of sugar in their blood (see insulin, oral diabetes medication).

Antigens: Substances that cause an immune response in the body, identifying substances or markers on cells; the body produces antibodies to fight antigens, or harmful substances, and tries to eliminate them.

Artery: A blood vessel that carries blood from the heart to other parts of the body; arteries are thicker than veins and have stronger, more elastic walls. Arteries sometimes develop plaque within their walls in a process known as "atherosclerosis." These plaques can become fragile and rupture, leading to complications associated with diabetes, such as heart attacks and strokes.

Artificial pancreas: A glucose sensor attached to an insulin delivery device; both are connected together by what is known as a "closed loop system." In other words, it is a system that not only can determine the body glucose level, but also takes that information and releases the appropriate amounts of insulin for the particular sugar it just measured.

Aspartame: An artificial sweetener used in place of sugar, because it has few calories; sold as "Equal" and "NutraSweet."

Asymptomatic: No symptoms; no clear sign that disease is present.

Atherosclerosis: A disease of the arteries caused by deposits of cholesterol in the walls of arteries; these plaques can build up and cause narrowing of the arteries or they can become fragile and break off, forming blood clots that cause heart attacks and stroke.

Autoimmune disease: A disorder of the body's immune system in which the immune system mistakenly attacks itself.

Autonomic neuropathy: Nerve damage to the part of the nervous system that we cannot consciously control; these nerves control our digestive system, blood vessels, urinary system, skin, and sex organs. Autonomic nerves are not under a person's control and function on their own.

Background retinopathy: This is the mildest form of eye disease caused by diabetes; it can be associated with normal vision. With a longer duration of diabetes or with uncontrolled blood sugars, eye damage can progress to more serious forms.

Basal rate: The amount of insulin required to manage normal daily blood glucose fluctuations; most people constantly produce insulin to manage the glucose fluctuations that occur during the day. In a person with diabetes, giving a constant low level amount of insulin via insulin pump mimics this normal phenomenon.

Beta cell: A type of cell in an area of the pancreas called the islets of Langerhans; beta cells make and release insulin, which helps control the glucose level in the blood.

Biosynthetic insulin: Genetically engineered human insulin; this insulin has a much lower risk of inducing an allergic reaction in people who use it, unlike cow (bovine) or pork (porcine) insulins. The manufacturers of synthetic insulin make it in a short-acting form, which works to cover mealtime increases in sugars; they also produce longer-acting insulins, which cover sugars between meals and when fasting, such as during the night.

Blood glucose: See glucose.

Blood glucose monitoring or testing: A method of testing how much sugar is in your blood; home blood-glucose monitoring involves pricking your finger with a lancing device, putting a drop of blood on a test strip and inserting the test strip into a blood-glucose-testing meter that displays your blood glucose level. Blood-sugar testing can also be done in the laboratory. Blood-glucose monitoring is recommended three or four times a day for people with insulin-dependent diabetes. Depending on the situation, glucose checks before meals, two hours after meals, at bedtime, in the middle of the night, and before and after exercise, may be recommended.

Blood pressure: The measurement of the pressure or force of blood against the blood vessels (arteries); blood pressure is written as two numbers. The first number or top number is called the systolic pressure and is the measure of pressure in the arteries when the heart beats and pushes more blood into the arteries. The second number, called the diastolic pressure, is the pressure in the arteries when the heart rests between beats. The ideal blood pressure for non-pregnant people with diabetes is 130/80 or less.

Brittle diabetes: When a person's blood sugar level often shifts very quickly from high to low and from low to high.

Blood urea nitrogen (BUN): A product of metabolism that is excreted in the urine; it is measured in the blood as an indirect measure of how well the kidney is functioning. Increased BUN levels in the blood may indicate early kidney damage, meaning the kidneys aren't effectively excreting BUN.

Bunion: Bump or bulge on the first joint of the big toe caused by the swelling of a sac of fluid under the skin and abnormalities in the joint; women are usually affected because of tight fitting or pointed shoes or high heels that put pressure on the toes, forcing the outward movement of the joint. People with flat feet or low arches are also prone to bunions. Shoes that fit well and are padded can prevent bunions from forming. Bunions may lead to other problems, such as serious infection from the big toe putting pressure on other toes.

Callus: A small area of skin, usually on the foot, that has become thick and hard from rubbing or pressure; calluses may lead to other problems, such as serious infection. Shoes that fit well can prevent calluses from forming.

Calorie: Energy that comes from food; some foods have more calories than others. Fats have more calories than proteins and carbohydrate. Most vegetables have few.

Carbohydrate: One of the three main classes of foods and a source of energy; carbohydrates are mainly sugars and starches that the body breaks down into glucose (a simple sugar that the body can use to feed its cells).

Cardiologist: A doctor who takes care of people with heart disease; a heart specialist.

Cardiovascular: Relating to the heart and blood vessels (arteries, veins, and capillaries).

Cholesterol: A waxy, odorless substance made by the liver that is an essential part of cell walls and nerves; cholesterol plays an important role in body functions such as digestion and hormone production. In addition to being produced by the body, cholesterol comes from animal foods that we eat. Too much cholesterol in the blood causes an increase in particles called LDL ("bad" cholesterol), which increases the buildup of plaque in the artery walls and leads to atherosclerosis.

Claudication: See intermittent claudication.

Coma: An emergency in which a person is not conscious; may occur in people with diabetes because their blood sugar is too high or too low.

Dawn phenomenon: A rise in blood sugar levels in the early morning hours.

Dehydration: Large loss of body water; if a person with diabetes has a very high blood sugar level, it causes increased water loss through increased urination and therefore, extreme thirst.

Diabetic ketoacidosis (DKA): A severe, life-threatening condition that results from hyperglycemia (high blood sugar), dehydration, and acid buildup that needs emergency fluid and insulin treatment; DKA happens when there is not enough insulin and cells become starved for sugars. An alternative source of energy called ketones becomes activated. The system creates a buildup of acids. Ketoacidosis can lead to coma and even death.

Dietitian: An expert in nutrition who helps people plan the type and amount of foods to eat for special health needs; a registered dietitian (RD) has special qualifications.

Emergency medical identification: Cards, bracelets, or necklaces with a written message, used by people with diabetes or other medical problems to alert others in case of a medical emergency, such as coma.

Endocrinologist: A doctor who treats people with hormone problems.

Exchange lists: A way of grouping foods together to help people on special diets stay on the diet; each group lists food in a serving size. A person can exchange, trade, or substitute a food serving in one group for another food serving in the same group. The lists put foods into six groups: starch/bread, meat, vegetables, fruit, milk, and fats. Within a food group, one serving of each food item in that group has about the same amount of carbohydrate, protein, fat, and calories.

Fasting plasma glucose test (FPG): The preferred method of screening for diabetes; the FPG measures a person's blood sugar level after fasting or not eating anything for at least 8 hours. Normal fasting blood glucose is less than 100 milligrams per deciliter or mg/dL. A fasting plasma glucose greater than 100 mg/dL and less than126 mg/dL implies that the person has an impaired fasting glucose level but may not have diabetes. A diagnosis of diabetes is made when the fasting blood glucose is greater than 126 mg/dL and when blood tests confirm abnormal results. These tests can be repeated on a subsequent day or by measuring glucose 2 hours after a meal. The results should show elevated blood glucose of more than 200 mg/dL.

Fats: Substances that help the body use some vitamins and keep the skin healthy; they are also the main way the body stores energy. In food, there are many types of fats -- saturated, unsaturated, polyunsaturated, monounsaturated, and trans-fats. To maintain your blood cholesterol and triglyceride (lipid) levels as near the normal ranges as possible, the American Diabetes Association recommends limiting the amount of saturated fats and cholesterol in our diets. Saturated fats contribute to blood levels of LDL ("bad") cholesterol. The amount of saturated fats should be limited to less than 10% of total caloric intake, and the amount of dietary cholesterol should be limited to 300 mg/day.

Fructose: A type of sugar found in many fruits and vegetables and in honey; fructose is used to sweeten some diet foods, but this type of sweetener is typically not recommended for people with diabetes, because it could have a negative effect on blood sugar.

Gangrene: The death of body tissues, usually due to a lack of blood supply, especially in the legs and feet.

Gastroparesis: A form of nerve damage that affects the stomach and intestines; with this condition, food is not digested properly and does not move through the stomach and intestinal tract normally. It can result in nausea and vomiting, because the transit time of food is slowed by nerve damage. This type of nerve damage can also cause a significant problem with low and erratic blood sugars.

Gestational diabetes: A high blood sugar level that starts or is first recognized during pregnancy; hormone changes during pregnancy affect the action of insulin, resulting in high blood sugar levels. Usually, blood sugar levels return to normal after childbirth. However, women who have had gestational diabetes are at increased risk of developing type II diabetes later in life. Gestational diabetes can increase complications during labor and delivery and increase the rates of fetal complications related to the increased size of the baby.

Glaucoma: An eye disease associated with increased pressure within the eye; glaucoma can damage the optic nerve and cause impaired vision and blindness.

Glucagon: A hormone that raises the level of glucose in the blood by releasing stored glucose from the liver; glucagon is sometimes injected when a person has lost consciousness (passed out) from low blood sugar levels. The injected glucagon helps raise the level of glucose in the blood.

Glucose: A simple sugar found in the blood; it is the body's main source of energy; also known as "dextrose."

Glucose tolerance test: A test to determine if a person has diabetes; the test is done in a lab or doctor's office in the morning before the person has eaten. A period of at least 8 hours without any food is recommended prior to doing the test. First, a sample of blood is taken in the fasting state. Then the person drinks a liquid that has sugar in it. Two hours later, a second blood test is done. A fasting blood sugar equal to or greater than 126 mg/dl is considered diabetes. A fasting blood sugar between 100 mg/dl and 125 mg/dl is classified as impaired fasting glucose. If the two-hour test result shows a blood sugar equal to or greater than 200 mg/dl, the person is considered to have diabetes. A two-hour blood glucose between 140 mg/dl and 199 mg/dl is classified as impaired glucose tolerance.

Glycated hemoglobin test (HbA1c): This is an important blood test to determine how well you are managing your diabetes; hemoglobin is a substance in red blood cells that carries oxygen to tissues. It can also attach to sugar in the blood, forming a substance called glycated hemoglobin or a Hemoglobin A1C. The test provides an average blood sugar measurement over a 6- to 12-week period and is used in conjunction with home glucose monitoring to make treatment adjustments. The ideal range for people with diabetes is generally less than 7%. This test can also be used to diagnose diabetes when the HbA1c level is equal to or greater than 6.5%.

High blood pressure: A condition when the blood flows through the blood vessels at a force greater than normal; high blood pressure strains the heart, harms the arteries, and increases the risk of heart attack, stroke, and kidney problems; also called "hypertension." The goal for blood pressure in people with diabetes is less than 130/80.

High blood sugar: See hyperglycemia.

Home blood glucose monitoring: A way in which a person can test how much sugar is in the blood; also called "self-monitoring of blood glucose." Home glucose monitoring tests whole blood (plasma and blood cell components); thus, the results can be different from lab values, which test plasma values of glucose. Typically, the lab plasma values can be higher than the glucose checks done at home with a glucose monitor.

Hormone: A chemical released in one organ or part of the body that travels through the blood to another area, where it helps to control certain bodily functions; for instance, insulin is a hormone made by the beta cells in the pancreas and when released, it triggers other cells to use glucose for energy.

Human insulin: Bio-engineered insulin very similar to insulin made by the body; the DNA code for making human insulin is put into bacteria or yeast cells and the insulin made is purified and sold as human insulin.

Hyperglycemia: High blood sugar; this condition is fairly common in people with diabetes. Many things can cause hyperglycemia. It occurs when the body does not have enough insulin or cannot use the insulin it does have.

Hypertension: See high blood pressure.

Hypoglycemia: Low blood sugar; the condition often occurs in people with diabetes. Most cases occur when there is too much insulin and not enough glucose in your body.

Impotence: Also called "erectile dysfunction;" persistent inability of the penis to become erect or stay erect. Some men may become impotent after having diabetes for a long time, because nerves and blood vessels in the penis become damaged. It is estimated that 50% of men diagnosed with type II diabetes experiences impotence.

Injection site rotation: Changing the areas on the body where a person injects insulin; by changing the area of injection, the injections will be easier, safer, and more comfortable. If the same injection site is used over and over again, hardened areas, lumps, or indentations can develop under the skin, which keep the insulin from being used properly. These lumps or indentations are called "lipodystrophies."

Injection sites: Places on the body where people can inject insulin most easily.

Insulin: A hormone produced by the pancreas that helps the body use sugar for energy; the beta cells of the pancreas make insulin.

Insulin mixture: A mixture of insulin that contains short-, intermediate- or long-acting insulin; you can buy premixed insulin to eliminate the need for mixing insulin from two bottles.

Insulin pump: A small, computerized device -- about the size of a small cell phone -- that is worn on a belt or put in a pocket; insulin pumps have a small flexible tube with a fine needle on the end. The needle is inserted under the skin of the abdomen and taped in place. A carefully measured, steady flow of insulin is released into the body.

Insulin reaction: Another term for hypoglycemia in a person with diabetes; this occurs when a person with diabetes has injected too much insulin, eaten too little food, or has exercised without eating extra food.

Insulin receptors: Areas on the outer part of a cell that allow insulin in the blood to join or bind with the cell; when the cell and insulin bind together, the cell can take glucose from the blood and use it for energy.

Insulin resistance: When the effect of insulin on muscle, fat, and liver cells becomes less effective; this effect occurs with both insulin produced in the body and with insulin injections. Therefore, higher levels of insulin are needed to lower the blood sugar.

Ketones: When the body starts to break down fat in order to get energy, ketones are a byproduct. When too many of those build up in the blood, it makes the blood acidic and can lead to diabetic ketoacidosis.

Lipohyertrophy: Lipohyertrophy occurs when an injection site is overused. The skin swells and a node can develop. The skin swells and may become tough. Injected insulin may not be absorbed very well from a site that has been overused.

Macrovascular complications: Over time, poor blood glucose control can lead to serious complications, including damage to major blood vessels — to the macrovascular system. Macrovascular complications cause plaque to build up in the arteries, which can lead to a heart attack, which can lead to a heart attack or stroke.

Microvascular complications: Over time, poor blood glucose control can lead to serious complications, including damage to tiny blood vessels — to the microvascular system. These microvascular complications of diabetes can lead to problems with the eyes (retinopathy or cataracts), kidneys (nephropathy), and nerves (neuropathy).

Nephropathy: Nephropathy is damage to the kidneys. It is a possible long-term complication of diabetes. *Nephr-* is a Greek root that means *kidney*, and *–pathy* is a Greek root meaning *damage*.

Neuropathy: Neuropathy is damage to the nerves. It is a possible long-term complication of diabetes. *Neuro-* is a Greek root that means *nerves*, and *–pathy* is a Greek root meaning *damage*.

Oral glucose tolerance test: The oral glucose tolerance test is one way that diabetes is diagnosed. It measures the blood glucose level five times over a period of three hours after you drink a high glucose mixture.

Pancreas: The pancreas is an organ of the endocrine system. A specific area of the pancreas, the islets of Langerhans, produces the hormone insulin.

Pre-diabetes: Pre-diabetes, also called glucose intolerance, is when a person has high blood glucose levels, but they aren't high enough *yet* to be diagnosed as diabetes. Pre-diabetes is an early sign of type II diabetes. Insulin resistance (when the body doesn't use insulin as well as it should) is another pre-diabetes sign.

Protein: Protein is a source of energy (as are carbohydrates and fat). Protein is found mainly in meat and beans.

Retinopathy: Retinopathy is damage to the retina. It is a possible long-term complication of diabetes. The retina is the part of the eye that senses light, and *–pathy* is a Greek root meaning *damage*.

Target range: Blood glucose levels need to stay within a certain range, and when you have diabetes, you must regulate your blood glucose levels with diet, exercise, and (perhaps) insulin. Before meals, the target range is 70 to 130mg/dL, and one to two hours after a meal, the target range is below 180mg/dL.

Chapter One: Understanding Type II Diabetes

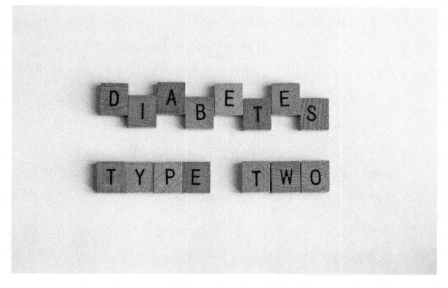

Before we delve deeper into what Type II diabetes is all about, it's imperative to know the basic facts of the bigger picture. We'll briefly discussed diabetes, some general facts, causes, symptoms and of course, its types so that you can further understand the condition in general.

As mentioned earlier, diabetes had been around since the ancient times. Back then Egyptians noticed that if your urine attracts the ants (or your urine is 'sweet'), that means there's something wrong with your system.

Of course, they had no idea what causes it or what this condition really means. We'll further discuss the history later on in this chapter.

Diabetes Mellitus is still one of the most common medical syndromes that people face today. This condition has a classification of two types, there's Type 1 diabetes and Type II diabetes. Type 1 is basically a syndrome in which the pancreatic cells that produce insulin are almost completely wiped out; type II is usually a dysfunction of these cells, to the point where the cells are no longer able to produce insulin that is effective in reducing glucose in the plasma.

The reasons for having type 1 diabetes are usually immune – mediated or in other words, your body's immune system attacks the pancreas itself, and so the cells that produce insulin are no longer able to produce insulin. For type II diabetes, it is usually weight - related or genetically - related issue; people who have a family history of the diseases usually have a higher instance of diabetes which is related to type II.

People who were diagnose with either type 1 and type II requires medication, however, with type 1 diabetes, medication starts almost immediately. Most people don't usually see any signs of symptoms, and if ever there's any, the symptoms are often very subtle and therefore hardly noticeable.

You will know for sure if you have diabetes once you've done blood tests. There are four different criteria for diabetes. The first one is, if your glucose or sugar levels are 126 or higher, you are considered diabetic (first stage). The second criteria is your protein marker called hemoglobin A1C, which is a protein that measures a three month interval of your past glucose averages; if your hemoglobin A1C is considered 6.6 or higher that means you are diabetic. The third indication is the obvious symptoms which are excessive or rapid weight loss, excessive thirst, frequent urination, blurry vision, headaches, dizziness, and fatigue. These symptoms along your blood glucose level measuring up to 200 can deemed you as diabetic. The last one is a two hour glucose test, if your blood sample measures 200 or more then you are again considered diabetic.

The American Diabetic Association recommends that individuals who are 45 years or older especially those who have a body mass index of 25 or higher, must be screened at least every 3 years to detect diabetes especially if there are no prevailing symptoms. If your family has a history of the disease, then it's highly recommended that you should be screened earlier to prevent and managed the disease.

Facts about Type II Diabetes

Now that you have a general idea or a brief overview of what diabetes is all about, we will now focused on one of the major types of diabetes' that has been a large contributing factor in many diseases today. In this section, you'll be given an overview of what Type II diabetes is all about including some of its causes, symptoms, and management; you can also find further information about each topic in succeeding chapters. We'll also bust some myths about type II diabetes so that you'll have a better perspective on how to deal with this illness.

As mentioned earlier, type II diabetes is the most common form of the disease, affecting almost 90% of patients worldwide.

Type II diabetes means that the body is unable to use insulin properly that is why it is also referred to as "insulin – resistant diabetes." In the beginning the pancreas might try to hold up and extract insulin but overtime what happens is that the pancreas will be unable to produce insulin to keep the blood sugar levels normal. When these happen, the sugar then will start to build up in the blood which will lead to high blood sugar levels. It is different from type 1 diabetes because there is an absolute lack of insulin because of the damage to the cells in the pancreas which produces insulin.

There are lots of reasons or factors that contribute to type II diabetes but more often than not the major causes are obesity and genetics; according to researchers, these are the strongest contenders of type II diabetes. The simplest way (and probably the most cliché advice) to prevent diabetes or type II diabetes for this matter is none other than leading a healthy lifestyle – that means keeping a tab on your diet and you should regularly exercise to stay fit because it can ultimately delay and in some cases, prevent the onset of diabetes.

Type 1 diabetes is quite easy to treat and managed compared to type II, because the former only needs to be injected with insulin, but the latter is a bit different and perhaps quite complicated. Initially, physicians will recommend regular monitoring of your blood sugar levels and will encourage you to eat a healthy diet, but if that doesn't work out, you may need to take medications, and for some people, especially those who are obese, may need to undergo a weight loss surgery. Type II diabetes is much more progressive than type 1, and if not treated properly or at an early stage, it can lead to serious complications and illnesses.

Myths and Facts

There are also lots of myths about people with type II diabetes, in this section, we will bust those myths out for you and give you nothing but facts.

Myth #1: Diabetes is not a serious illness

If you think diabetes is not serious then you'll be dead before you know it! Diabetes alone can't ultimately kill you but it will cause other serious complications such as cardiovascular diseases and even stroke. If you don't prevent it or take proper measures, you'll surely fall into its trap.

Myth #2: You'll automatically have type II diabetes if you are overweight or obese.

Well, this is not entirely true, although as we've mentioned earlier, obesity is one of the major factors that come into play but it doesn't mean that you'll automatically get the disease once you gain some pounds. A lot of factors such as family history or genetics as well as having high blood pressure or hypertension can cause you to acquire the disease.

Myth #3: Being detected with diabetes means that your body is not producing insulin

That's a myth because all human beings produce insulin! Patients who have type II diabetes on their first diagnosis usually have normal insulin levels, however, it comes to a point where insulin can no longer cause cells in the body to absorb sugar from food, that's when the pancreas stops producing enough insulin to keep the blood sugar levels down or to a normal range. Once this happens, the patient will eventually have type II diabetes.

Myth #4: You don't need to test blood sugar levels because you can feel it when you have high blood sugar or low blood sugar

First of all, if you are diabetic, it's required that you monitor your sugar levels from time to time. You just can't rely with how you feel or the present symptoms you were experiencing. If you have been regarded as diabetic, these symptoms or feelings will get less accurate over time. You may feel dizzy or lightheaded when you have low levels of sugar or you can experience a flu or bladder infection when you have high levels of sugar but you'll never know for sure unless you get tested.

Myth #5: Diabetic people is prohibited in eating sweets

This is perhaps the most popular or recognized idea that immediately comes to people's mind once someone is diagnosed with diabetes. Patients with type II diabetes or even type 1 diabetes can still eat sweets as long as it fits one's normal meal plan and if it is properly distributed with healthy foods. However, like any other diseases, you need to take it in moderation, since uncontrolled levels of sugar in the blood is the main problem with diabetic patients, you need to make sure that you just have enough sugar and not too much of it. Desserts and soft drinks contain lots of sugar which can spike glucose levels in the bloodstream; it can wreak havoc to your blood which can cause a problem. The main point here is that you can eat sweet, just make sure to balance it within your diet.

A Brief History of Diabetes

Diabetes is one of the longest and deadliest "silent killer" diseases ever known to mankind. Understanding how our ancestors from previous centuries discovered it and managed it, ultimately led us to where we are today. Let's take a look at the brief history of how science and medicine helped patients combat the disease over the years.

600 BC: Early Egyptians discovered a condition where a person has "honey urine."

400 – 500 BC: Indian physicians Sushruta and Charaka first identified the difference between type 1 and type II diabetes. They associated type 1 with youth and type II with overweight people.

200 BC: Demetrius of Apamea from Greece first coined the term "diabetes."

100 AD: Aretaeus of Cappadocia described diabetes for the first time ever.

1000: For the first time in human history, a scientist described the taste of the sweet urine or honey urine.

1792: Diabetes Mellitus and Diabetes Insipidus was differentiated by JP Frank.

1807: Chevreul found out that glucose was the sugar present in the sweet urine

1855: Claude Bernard introduced the term glycogen (glucose maker) and coined the term internal secretion where he discovered the secretion of glucose or sugar in the blood stream.

1921 – 1922: Canadian physicists, Frederick Banting and Charles Best, finally isolated and purified insulin

1940 – Present: The NPH Insulin was further developed to help control blood sugar levels among diabetic patients. Diagnosis, management, medicines and alternative treatments were further studied and developed to help people combat the disease.

Chapter Two: Types of Type II Diabetes

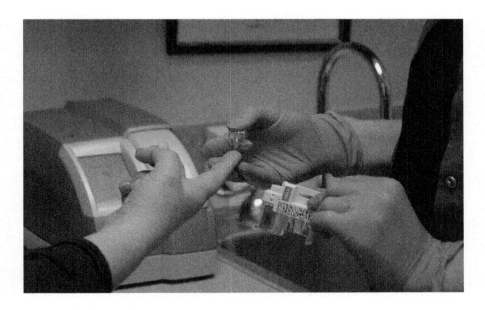

You now know that there are two major types of diabetes – type 1 and type II, as a matter of fact, there are three, but the third one is only exclusive for pregnant women, it's called gestational diabetes. Not a lot of patients know that type II can be classified into four more types or sub – types. The classifications in this chapter are not official but some physicians and researchers agreed that it is under the category of type II diabetes. This might broaden your knowledge further and could also help you in possibly identifying which category you fall into so you can act accordingly.

Sub – Types or Categories of Type II Diabetes

According to some researchers, type II diabetes can be classified into four; these are type O, type I, subtype H, and subtype S. In this section, we'll briefly discuss these subtypes and also provide some general guideline on what to do or what you should avoid to be able to control or at least manage it.

- **Type O**

According to studies, type O is pretty much a classic type II diabetes. Around 50 – 60% of patients are overweight and are highly insulin resistant. Most patients have off – the charts insulin levels (which means that the body is uncontrollably producing excess insulin) and usually, it is often too late once the patients found out. The symptoms are very subtle, that's why if you are overweight, or have a family history of the disease you should test your blood sugar levels every now and then.

- **Type I**

Type I is referred to as the "thin or mild version" of type II diabetes. Patients who were diagnosed with type II diabetes that belongs to the type I category could be underweight and have very low levels of insulin but they have high levels of glucose in their bloodstream. These patients are often diagnose specifically with Latent Autoimmune Diabetes of Adults (LADA). Type I patients should only have small frequent feeding so that their low levels of insulin can handle and control the glucose in the bloodstream. Low carb foods and a small chunk of protein should be their ideal diet.

- **Subtype H**

H stands for hormonal, patients classified under subtype H often have worn out adrenal glands and they usually have low thyroid. These patients could be slightly overweight or even have a normal weight but their bodies could get easily inflamed. Patients under subtype H may or may not be insulin resistant as well. If you fall under this category you may need carbs (although it may not work for some depending on your current condition and other factors) but since the adrenal glands cannot produce enough carbs, the patient needs to compensate for that lack through incorporating carbohydrate rich foods in their diet. Some examples are sweet potatoes or beets (best for people who can't easily sleep).

- **Subtype S**

S stands for stress – induced, your type II diabetes can either be caused by long – term chronic stress or one big time traumatic stress. Patients under this subcategory have, obviously, high levels of stress hormones or cortisol and adrenaline in their body which then causes an increase in blood sugar levels. If you think you are under this classification, then better eat up some carbs (but not too much though) and also limit caffeine and alcohol or any other similar stimulants. You can also try some supplements but consult your doctor first before taking any.

Another important not is that, if you fall in this subtype, exercise may not be suitable for you because once you do; your body will release cortisol which in turn would raise your sugar levels, instead of going down. However, that doesn't mean that you should not exercise anymore! You can still do some light exercises such as yoga or tai chi to help your body combat the disease.

Chapter Three: Progression of Type II Diabetes

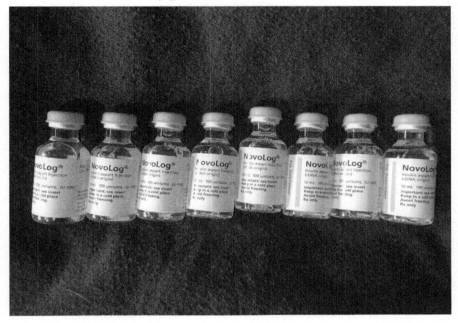

Type II diabetes is a naturally progressive disease, as a matter of fact, once the patient is finally diagnosed with type II diabetes, many changes have probably occurred in the body; it could already trigger heart disease and may have affected the functioning of some organs. These subtle changes will continue over time, making the complications much more difficult to manage and control (especially if the patient has other current or underlying illnesses). In this chapter, you'll be given an overview on what to expect once you found out that you have type II diabetes so that you can prepare for your health and be able to manage it ahead of time.

Phases and Process of Type II Diabetes

According to many experts, once a patient is officially diagnosed with type II diabetes, they may actually already have diabetes – related problems long before they know it! Chances are the buildup of high glucose levels in the blood stream already caused some damage to your kidneys, heart and nerves way before noticeable symptoms appear. So if you are "newly" diagnosed, that means you have been "in the club" long before you realize it.

So what happens next? After finding out, your pancreas may still not know that there's a problem because as tests will show, it will still produce normal amounts of insulin in the body in order to keep blood sugar or glucose under control. But overtime, the cells will eventually resist the insulin – which means that you've now entered level 2, doctors called it "insulin resistance." Once your cells can't no longer use the naturally occurring insulin; your pancreas will then be "notified," and to overcome this resistance, it will begin to produce more insulin than before. At some point, it will not be able to keep up with the body's high demands, and sugar levels in your bloodstream will continue to increase. This phase is now called pre – diabetes. It's like your almost there but not quite!

Pre-diabetes means that your blood sugar is higher than normal, but may not be high enough to be classified as diabetes. Now, once you've reached this stage, there's still a chance to at least delay it or prevent yourself from actually being diagnosed as diabetic. According to many physicians, this is the time to really consider losing weight (if you are overweight) or eating a balanced diet food and regularly exercising a few minutes each day because it helps lower blood pressure, improve blood fats, and also reduce the risk of heart diseases. It is in this phase where your pancreas tries to produce insane amounts of insulin rapidly. Think of it as "panic mode." You can help your pancreas calm down by eating good nutrition and waking up your immune system through exercise.

If for some reason, you didn't try your best to prevent from progressing to the diabetic stage or if it's already too late; your pancreas will be "burnt out," in producing insulin and it will eventually begin to wear out. Once this happens, your sugar levels will now increase and you will officially be classified as a diabetic. Welcome to the club!

When you've reached this point, that means that your pancreas has already lost 50% of its ability to produce insulin. Aside from a balanced diet and regular exercise, you will then be prescribed with one or two types of medicines. Most likely, your physician will prescribe one pill to increase production of insulin, and another pill to decrease the cell's resistance to insulin. However, since your pancreas will continue to decline in its ability to produce insulin, many patients diagnosed with type II are eventually advised to take insulin.

As blood sugar goes out of control and your disease progresses, you and your doctor needs to work together especially when it comes to monitoring and keeping tab on your sugar levels. You will be advised to take in proper nutrition, take appropriate meds and match it all with a physical activity that is suitable for you. The key to control your blood glucose is regular monitoring and of course, following your physician's advice or suggestion.

Chapter Four: Causes, Diagnosis, and Treatment

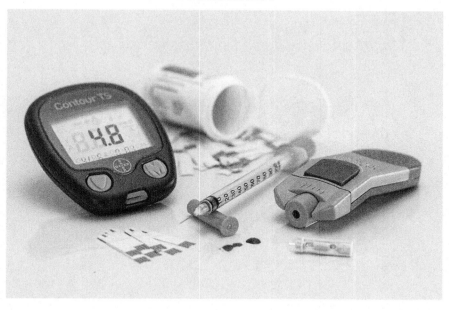

Now that you have an overview of what type II diabetes is, its types and how it can affect one's physical health, it's now time to get into the details. In this chapter you will be given a depth of information about its various causes, common symptoms, diagnosis, and risk factors, as well as various options for medical treatment. Knowing the enemy inside out will help prevent you from doing the wrong things that could worsen your condition. If you have enough knowledge about what causes it or the symptoms you need to watch out for, you may have a bigger chance of making a change for yourself.

Major Causes of Type II Diabetes

Type II diabetes has many other related causes such as lifestyle factors, but in this section, we'll focus first on the usual causes of how a pre – diabetic person progresses to being diabetic.

Obesity, Overweight and Lack of Exercise

Obesity or being way above the normal weight is one of the major causes of type II diabetes. If you have read the first chapter of this book, you may remember that early Indian scientists associated type II diabetes with being overweight - now that says a lot! Because back then even if they haven't figured everything out yet, even if the field of medicine is not yet advanced, and most of the time they are only relying on observation, these ancient physicians have pinpoint the exact same cause that scientists have proven today!

If you are overweight, you will most likely progress to having type II diabetes because an extra or I would say, an excess weight causes further insulin resistance. Your extra belly fat is also linked to insulin resistance and cardiovascular diseases. But if you think about it, it's not really obesity right? What I mean by that is, obesity or being overweight is already a result, so the main cause of why you'll have type II diabetes in the first place is simple: lack of regular exercise and balanced nutrition. In fact, all diseases boil down to that. This is the simplest and most practical advice that can ultimately make your body stronger and healthier, unfortunately though; lots of people take it for granted. Don't be one of them!

Genetics and Family History

Some medical research suggests that people diagnosed with type II diabetes have certain genes that tend to develop or increase the risk of being diagnosed as diabetic. The disease usually occurs among African Americans, Alaskan natives, Americans, Hispanics, and Pacific Islanders.

Like any other diseases or conditions, your genetic makeup can affect everything in your health, and most of the time if you have a certain kind of condition, a type II diabetes for this matter, you can traced it back to your family. If it's not in your immediate family, maybe your uncles or cousins or other relatives might have had it in the past. However, take note that people who were born in a family with a diabetic history don't usually inherit the condition (sometimes it will be pass down either to your kids or your grandkids); it's not absolute that if your parents or relatives are diabetic you will be automatically diabetic too. But it's more likely that you will if you don't eat right and stay fit.

Other Possible Causes

- **Cystic Fibrosis**

This occurs when a thick mucus is being produced in the pancreas which causes the organ to be scarred, once this happens, it can prevent the pancreas from making enough insulin that controls blood sugar.

- **Hemochromatosis**

It causes the body to store excessive amounts of iron, and if (pre) diabetes is not immediately treated, iron can accumulate which could damage the body's other organs including the pancreas.

- **Monogenic Diabetes**

This is caused by genetic mutation or a change in a single gene, it is usually inherited from families who have had previous history with diabetes but more often than not, it occurs on its own. This gene mutation causes the pancreas to not properly function and produce lesser amounts of insulin in the body.

Here are the two common type of monogenic diabetes:

- **Neonatal Diabetes:** Common among newborns within the first six months.
- **Maturity – Onset Diabetes (MODY):** occurs during adolescence or early adulthood, although sometimes it is detected later in life.

- **Hormonal Diseases**

Hormonal diseases can cause the body to produce too much hormones that affects the production of insulin and the absorption of blood sugar into the cells. Here are some examples of hormonal diseases that can cause diabetes:

- **Crushing Syndrome:** Causes the body to produce too much cortisol or otherwise known as the "stress hormone."
- **Acromegaly:** happens when the body produces excessive growth hormone.
- **Hyperthyroidism:** happens when the body produces excessive thyroid hormones that can affect the cells and insulin production.

- **Pancreatitis**

Diseases related to pancreas such as pancreatic cancer or any pancreatic trauma can affect the beta cells in the pancreas and cause it to produce less insulin. If the pancreas is removed or replaced, diabetes can also occur due to loss of beta cells.

- **Medicines**

Meds especially for those who have other illnesses can also have side – effects and could disrupt beta cells and insulin production which could increase the chance of diabetes. This includes the following:

- Niacin
- Water pills
- Anti-seizure drugs
- Psychiatric drugs
- drugs to treat HIV
- Pentamidine (for pneumonia)
- Glucocorticoids (for inflammatory ilnnesses)
- Anti-rejection medicines (for transplanted organ)
- Statins (for bad cholesterol/ LDL)

Symptoms of Type II Diabetes

As you may now know, the symptoms especially at a very early stage are very subtle, you may not notice it and even if you already have high levels of blood sugar, you may still not feel a single thing. Noticing subtle changes in your body can be very helpful in preventing further damage of the disease, you should watch out for the following symptoms:

- Frequent urination and increased in thirst
- Increased hunger
- Fatigue or too much stress
- Blurry vision
- Numbness of feet and hands
- Sores that doesn't heal quickly
- Unexplained weight loss

Keep in mind that diabetic people diagnosed as type II usually have had these symptoms already but it's so mild that one can hardly notice it, because this kind of diabetes progresses at a very slow rate over the course of many years. It's highly recommended that if any of your family had the disease, you should look out for subtle changes.

Risk Factors

The progression rate of type II diabetes may likely develop at a much rapid pace if it is combined with other risk factors. While you can't change your genetic makeup, age, ethnicity and family history, your lifestyle choices and other health conditions can ultimately affect your chances of having diabetes. Here are the risk factors for diabetics with type II condition:

- If you are 45 years old and above
- If you have hypertension or high blood pressure
- If you have high levels of tryglicerides and low levels of "good cholesterol" or HDL
- If you gave birth to more than a 9 pound baby and has a history of gestational diabetes (for pregnant women); it can progress to type II.
- If you have experienced heart attacks or stroke before
- If you previously had depressive episodes (mental condition, not just a one – time depression)
- If you have polycystic ovary syndrome (PCOS)
- If you have a dark, velvety thick skin around your neck called *acanthosis nigricans* (common among obese people or overweight people).

Diagnosis

If you think you or any of your friends and family has been experiencing some signs of diabetes, you may want to consult a psychologist or seek medical help as soon as you can. If potential diabetic patients are diagnosed at an early stage and was given treatment as soon as possible, you'd be able to deal with it and manage its effects. People who seek professional help live very normal lives.

As previously mentioned in the progression chapter of this book, you are not yet considered diabetic if you haven't hit the target or official level of glucose in your blood stream but of course, you will eventually get to that stage if you don't get diagnosed early on.

Physicians recommend routine testing for type II diabetes if you are 45 years and above, if you are overweight (especially at a young age) and if you are a woman who recently just gave birth and had a history of gestational diabetes. Aside from that, doctors also advise routine checkup for obese kids between the ages of 10 and 18 as well as kids who had a low birth weight or if the mother had diabetes while she was pregnant with the child.

The kind of test that doctors usually implement to detect if you are predisposed to diabetes or positive of the disease is called the Hemoglobin A1C test, also referred to as HbA1c or Glycohemoglobin test. The test simply provides information about the average blood glucose level for the 3 – month period. It is the primary test for diabetes management and research. It will pretty much tell you on what stage you are (either pre-diabetic or diabetic stage).

Important Note

Your physician may advise you to take other types of test for accuracy purposes (see chapter 1 for other types of test). Nevertheless, it's important to let your doctor or medical provider administer the test especially if you think you have the symptoms or would want a simple routine checkup. You should not just buy glucose test equipment at a drug store to see for yourself because more often than not it is inaccurate. Always seek professional help.

Treatment

Aside from eating healthy foods and taking proper exercise or physical activity, you will eventually be advised to take medications and of course insulin intake. In this section we'll discuss some methods on how to take insulin, oral medicines for diabetes as well as other injectable meds for you to be able to manage your type II diabetes as it progress from one phase to another.

Common Medications

Various kinds of diabetes medications are a big help to control, manage and treat type II diabetes. Physicians usually recommend diabetic patients an oral medication such as metformin pills. These pills are the "starter" pills, they are in liquid form, and can help your lower the blood glucose in your liver as well as help your body properly use the naturally occurring insulin. For slightly overweight patients, this drug could also help you lose some weight.

There are other diabetes medications that act in different ways to lower or control the rising levels of your blood sugar. Your doctor will most probably recommend one or two diabetic pills in combination with other treatment methods to help normalize the glucose in your bloodstream.

It's also important to always have a follow – up checkup with your doctor so that you can have a gauge if the current medication is working or not. Here are some guidelines before taking any diabetic oral medications:

Tips before taking any medication:

- Always talk to a legit doctor or pharmacist before taking any medication so that you should be aware of its effects and possible side – effects to the body.

- If there are any side – affects you should report it immediately to the doctor so that he or she can change the medicine or maybe give a more appropriate dosage.

- Don't suddenly stop taking any medication without first consulting your doctor, or combine it with other types of medicine. This could worsen your condition and the pill or medicine may not work properly if the scheduled or frequency of intake is not followed.

Important Note:

The medicine will vary depending on the type of your diabetes, the initial result once you take them, and also other factors including your current health condition. The daily schedule and dosage of the medicine prescribed will also play a role in your condition's improvement, so make sure you follow it.

Insulin

For patients who are just in the pre – diabetes stage, you may not yet be advised to take insulin as long as proper nutrition and exercise worked out, but if things didn't go well, your disease will naturally progress to a point where your body will not be producing enough insulin to help your cells absorbed blood sugar, which is why most patients starts to take in insulin. Insulin intake is a must if you are officially diagnosed as diabetic.

There are various methods in which you can take insulin; this may depend on your preference, lifestyle, insurance coverage, budget etc. The most common type of insulin intake is through needles but there are also other unique and probably better ways for different types of diabetic patients such as insulin pump, pen injections, inhalers, injection ports and jet injectors.

- **Needle and Syringe**

The most common type of insulin intake is through the needle and syringe. You can do an insulin shot to yourself or other person may administer it for you. Once you filled up your syringe with insulin from a vial or bottle you can inject it right in your belly, in your arm, in your thighs, or even your butt. Although according to most medical professionals, insulin works fastest when injected in the belly or on your tummy, just make sure to change the spots where you inject the insulin.

- **Insulin Pen**

Insulin pens work just like a needle and syringe, the only difference is that insulin pens already comes filled with insulin and has a needle. Unlike in ordinary injections, you need to fill up the syringe and manually put in the needle before taking the shot. Insulin pens are much easier to use and also portable. There are some versions where you can insert a cartridge (pre-filled with insulin) and just replace them with a new one after use. Insulin pens cost more than the traditional needle and syringe but most patients are now switching to it because of its convenience.

- **Pump**

    Some patients prefer an insulin pump. Insulin pumps are a small machine that gives patient steady doses of insulin shots in a day. You could wear it outside your body, hang it on your belt or put it in your inside pocket or pouch. The machine is connected to a small plastic tube with a small needle, and all you have to do is inject the needle on a particular spot under your skin where it will stay for a couple of days. The insulin will automatically be pumped through the tube in your body 24/7 so that you won't need to always remind yourself to have an insulin shot throughout the day. There are other versions where the pump is directly attached to your skin with no tubes like a self – adhesive pod.

- **Inhaler**

You can also take insulin by using an inhaler, although this is only recommended for adults with type 1 or type II diabetes. You just need to breathe the powdered insulin so that it will go straight to your lungs and can be absorbed quickly into your bloodstream.

- **Injection Port**

Injection port is one of the lesser methods used by diabetic patients. Injection ports have a short tube that you insert under your skin, and an adhesive patch is attached to it. The patch functions as a dressing and a port wherein you can inject yourself either using an insulin pen or a needle and syringe, the port will stay in place for a couple of days but of course, you need to replace at some point. The only advantage of using injection ports is that you will no longer puncture your skin every time you take an insulin shot.

- **Jet Injector**

Another less common method is using a jet injector. A jet injector is a high – tech device in which it will finely spray insulin into your skin at high levels of pressure without using a needle or puncturing yourself. This can be quite expensive but can also be convenient.

Here are the most common FDA approved insulin injectables:

- Basaglar (insulin glargine injection)
- Tresiba (insulin degludec injection)
- Ryzodeg (insulin aspart: insulin degludec)
- Toujeo (insulin glargine injection)
- Lucentis (ranibizumab)
- Glyxambidisclaimer (icon empagliflozin and linagliptin)
- Trulicitydisclaimer (icon duglaglutide)
- Invokametdisclaimer (icon canagliflozin and metformin hydrochloride)
- Jardiance (empagliflozin)
- Afrezza (Inhalation Powder insulin human)
- Tanzeum (abliglutide)
- Farxiga (dapaglifozin)
- Invokana (canagliflozin)
- Nesina (alogliptin benzoate)

There are other non – insulin injectable that your doctor might recommend, however it can cause hypoglycemia or low blood glucose. If you don't properly balanced your food with your medications, or if you don't follow the appropriate dosage and schedule intake, it might cause some side – effects. Non – insulin injectable medicines are not a substitute for insulin, make sure to ask your physician before taking anything to prevent side – effects and further worsen your condition.

Other Treatments:

- **Bariatric Surgery**

It is also known as metabolic surgery or weight – loss surgery. This procedure could help patients who are obese and diagnosed with type II diabetes through normalizing blood sugar levels in the body by removing excess fats.

- **Artificial Pancreas**

Artificial pancreas replaces manual blood sugar testing. This system monitors your blood sugar levels 24/7 and provides combination of insulin shots and glucagon automatically. The FDA recently approved a hybrid – closed loop system (a type of artificial pancreas) that monitors your glucose every 5 minutes and automatically gives your body insulin shot day and night. It eliminates the daily task of manually giving a shot to yourself or waking up at night just to see your blood sugar levels. This new artificial pancreas will be available in the U.S. in 2017.

Diabetic Emergencies

Diabetic patients may at one point or another experience an emergency; your blood sugar can either shoot up (hyperglycemia) or decline dramatically (hypoglycemia) in a short period of time. If you have excessive amounts of insulin, it could cause low glucose levels which means that you need a rush of insulin immediately, on the other hand, if there aren't enough insulin, it could cause high levels of blood sugar which means that you could potentially experience diabetic coma.

Here are the most common symptoms to look out for if you are or will be experiencing hypoglycemia:

- Sudden drowsiness or weakness
- Pale and sweaty skin
- Rapid pulse and breathing
- Headache, dizziness or trembling
- Numbness in both hands and feet
- Sudden hunger

- Odorless breath

Here are the most common symptoms to look out for if you are or will be experiencing hyperglycemia:

- Nausea
- Deep and sighing breaths
- Rapid pulse
- Confusion
- Unsteady gait
- Warm or flushed and dry skin
- Gradual loss of consciousness

First Aid

- If the person is unconscious or unresponsive, call 911 or emergency numbers of the nearest hospital ASAP.

- You can also in the meantime administer CPR while waiting for medical response. Make sure to place the person on a flat surface and check the breathing, pulse rate and circulation before performing CPR. Do not perform the procedure if you are not educated or haven't had any previous experience.

- If the person is conscious assist him or her in getting the right medications, or administer insulin shot (for hypoglycemia/low blood sugar patients only).

- If the person is disoriented, try to give him/her food or a drink, make him/her comfortable and immediately seek for medical assistance.

Chapter Five: Prevention and Management

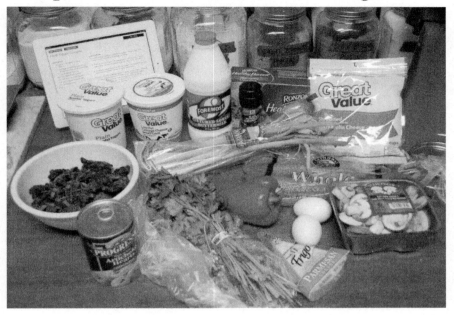

You will not choose to buy or read this book in the first place if you are not affected with the disease. Maybe you are diagnosed as a diabetic, or you have recently found out that your blood sugar is not normal or you might be overweight, perhaps your family and friends might be affected too which is why you wanted to learn more about the disease and how it could affect you or the ones you loved. In this chapter, you'll learn how to prevent (or delay) your condition and also manage diabetes so that you can at least make better choices and live healthier lives. Read on!

Preventing Type II Diabetes

Diabetes can cause other illnesses or if you already have one, it can worsen and affect your current condition. Type II diabetes can cause heart diseases, stroke, vision problems, and foot sores just to name a few. Even if you are still in the pre – diabetic stage, it could already start causing other illnesses. The longer you have diabetes, the higher chance you'll likely develop complications and other diseases.

Fortunately, type II diabetes or diabetes in general can be delayed and even prevented right before it kills you. Delaying it could be beneficial to you and your long-term health! Follow these simple yet most taken for granted tips so that you can stop diabetes before it starts destroying your body.

- **Lose Weight and Stay Fit!** (for obese/ overweight patients)

If you think that your weight is already above the normal range, then this is the time to really start shedding those excess pounds, not because you want to look good, but because you want to save your life! Even if you are just diagnosed as pre – diabetic, you can start losing at least 5 – 7 % of your starting weight to delay diabetes, so if for example, you weigh 150 pounds, your goal should at least lose about 10 pounds or more. Don't expect to lose weight easily, and don't force yourself or do drastic measures to shed a lot of pounds within a short period of time. It might take some time (depending on you) before you lose a pound or two. It will be easier said than done, so just take it easy, have some discipline and always focus on your goals.

- **Move, move, move!**

This advice goes is applicable to overweight, underweight or even patients who have normal weight. If you have a family history of diabetes, if you think you are experiencing subtle symptoms or if you notice that your blood sugar is increasing, then what are you waiting for? Move! Exercise! Do any physical activity that is suitable for you (ask your physician for a recommendation) because an active life can improve and awaken your immune system that can ultimately combat the disease! If you want to heal yourself naturally and also be able to keep a healthy and fit lifestyle, always be on the move!

You can actually start small; you don't have to sign up for a gym membership, or buy expensive equipment or even hire a professional trainer, just a simple walk around the park or on the street every day for at least 30 minutes to 1 hour can change your life!

- **Eat Like a human not a beast!**

It might sound harsh but it holds true for any diseases, if physicians or health professionals said it this way, it can most likely catch a patient's attention, probably remember it and take the advice very seriously. The idea behind this is that, humans are designed to eat veggies and foods that are soft.

If you'll notice the structure of a human's teeth, it is square and flat just like a goat or a cow, which means that it's created to chew on green or soft foods such as salads, fruits, veggies etc. On the other hand, the teeth of "beasts" or predators such as lions, tigers, bears, sharks among many have fangs or sharp teeth which mean that it is built to eat meat and foods that are hard to chew. However, humans seem to think they are "beasts," and most of us are guilty of eating foods that are not appropriate for our bodies.

The trick is to eat smaller portions of meat (you still need a healthy dose of protein), combine it with healthy dishes such as salads, and as much as possible avoid drinking soft drinks or sweetened beverages. You need to choose foods that have small caloric content, less sugar and foods that have built in vitamins and minerals which can be found in vegetables and fruits so that your body will absorb nothing but nutrients.

Managing Type II Diabetes

The key to managing diabetes and living a long, healthy and happy life lies on the choices you make each day. You may not be able to control variables like your age, your genes or the diseases you inherit from your family but you can still live a normal and healthy life if you will it!

If you have diabetes, your physician will recommend you to take medications and regularly monitor your blood sugar levels every single day; however, you also need to always check your cholesterol levels as well as blood pressure to prevent potential health problems in the future.

The most essential part for you to successfully manage your diabetic condition aside from closely monitoring your health is to work closely with your doctors, health care "team," and of course your loved ones. You're not alone in this battle; always remember that a lot of people are there to help you win the war!

Here are some tips on how to manage diabetes:

- **Always keep tab on your diabetic status**

This is a must but don't let your condition get in your head way too much. Don't be obsessed with the numbers, just be responsible on your stats and focus on getting better. If your doctor recommends you to take the hemoglobin A1C test, don't be afraid and take it, how can you successfully defeat the enemy if you don't know where you stand? These tests will help you plan the things you need to do to achieve your goal of controlling your diabetes. The usual A1C test goal for diabetics is 7% below; the goal when it comes to blood pressure is 140/90 mm Hg. Take control of your cholesterol and ask your physician on how to eliminate bad cholesterol so that it won't clog up your blood vessels which could lead to various heart conditions.

- **Stop smoking and avoid frequent alcohol consumption**

    Diabetes and bad cholesterol are not the only factors that clog up your blood vessel but also smoking. If your blood vessel clogs up, it will make your heart work harder which often leads to cardiovascular illnesses. E - Cigarettes are not good options either as well as frequent or excessive alcohol intake. You don't want to add more "enemies" or risk factors that could help enhance your diabetes and make it harder to manage. Here are some advantages for diabetics if they quit smoking:

    - You'll lower chances of various health problems including kidney diseases, respiratory diseases, nerve problems, stroke, eye and foot problems and even amputation.
    - It will improve your cholesterol and blood pressure
    - Your blood circulation will get better
    - You'll find exercising easier

- **Create and maintain your diabetic meal plan**

    The importance of good nutrition is very much emphasized in this book and I'm sure your doctor also recommends the same advice. You need to stop eating junk and start eating balanced diet that includes fruits, veggies, whole grains, chicken (without the skin), lean meat, fish, cheese, and low – fat milk. As much as possible avoid or completely stop drinking sweetened beverages and choose foods that are low in trans-fat, calories, saturated fat, sugar and salt.

Ask your physician on the appropriate diet plan for you, there is no exact or generic meal plan for diabetic patients because it will highly depend on your current condition and possible underlying illnesses. Make sure to follow and eat the right foods to boost your body functions.

- **Make sure to incorporate physical activities on your daily routine**

Swimming and brisk walking are good exercises for diabetic patients, you don't really need to do extreme exercises or excessive workouts, just make sure to not sit around all day and keep moving. You can ask your physicians on the best exercise you can do because it also depends on your age, risk factors and other conditions. You can also create a workout plan that'll go hand in hand with your diabetes meal plan.

- **Work with Your Health Care Team**

Make sure to always work with your health care team. If you are in the field of sports, in the field of business, and even in the field of medicine, you have to have the right people on your team to make win championships, to properly execute a world changing idea, or to simple save someone's life. You can't fight diabetes alone; in fact, you shouldn't fight it alone because chances are you may not get well easily and quickly if you have no "support system." Aside from your medical physician, and family members, some people who will be part of your "healthcare team" are the following:

- **Diabetologist** – he/she will serve as your consultant; a specialist and an expert who can ultimately help you treating the disease.

- **Diabetist Specialist Nurse** – Just like the diabetologist, he/she is specially trained to help patients in managing your condition.

- **Endocrinologist** – since diabetes is a progressive condition, your general physician will most likely recommend you getting another expert to keep track of your endocrine system (thyroid, adrenal, pituitary gland etc.), in order to make sure that other vital organs which can affect insulin production are regulated to prevent further complications.

- **Registered Dietitian** – you may also need a dietitian to help you plan your meals. You need to have a balanced diet with the proper ratio/amount for your body to fight diabetes and also strengthen your immune system. Aside from the ratio of food, your RD will give recommendations and help you choose the right foods to buy even after you've already been treated so that you can maintain your diet.

- **Eye Doctor/Podiatrist/Physiologist** – your diabetes may cause further complications that can affect your eyesight or vision, make you develop foot and sore problems and also make you obese. This is the reason why you need eye doctors, podiatrist (foot and sore problem specialist) and physiologist to help you control any common complications and keep you healthy.

- **Other Health Specialist** – this goes out for those patients who are diabetic with other illnesses like renal, cardiovascular, pancreatic, liver, intestinal diseases etc. You and your own specialist doctors will need to work hand in hand to control both diseases without creating conflicts in terms of medicines and procedures. Sometimes, meds have certain side effects to the body which could affect other vital organs which is why your doctors will most likely ask for approval first from your other specialist doctor (if you have other major illnesses) before prescribing you any medicine or doing any procedure.

- **Have a positive mindset, engage in positive activities, and live a happy life!**

Being diagnose with diabetes could be daunting for a lot of people, but what good will it bring you and your loved ones if you'll just focus on the problem instead of working towards the solution? If you can't prevent it, then manage it, try to deal with it and do your best to achieve your goals of living a healthier lifestyle. Aside from following the doctor's rules, you should also learn how to turn this problem around, think of it as an opportunity and work towards becoming a better version of yourself. Be positive about it and live as if you haven't been diagnosed with diabetes!

Try to join fun activities such as yoga, tai chi, meditation, and various community building causes or attend diabetic forums so that you and other patients can empower one another. Get enough sleep (7 - 8 hours every night), and reduce your stress levels by doing your favorite hobby, rocking out to your favorite music as well as spending time with your friends and family; this will not only improve your blood circulation but it will also revitalize your mind, body and soul! Oh and don't forget to laugh! Laughter is still the best medicine.

Chapter Six: Alternative Treatment for Type II Diabetes

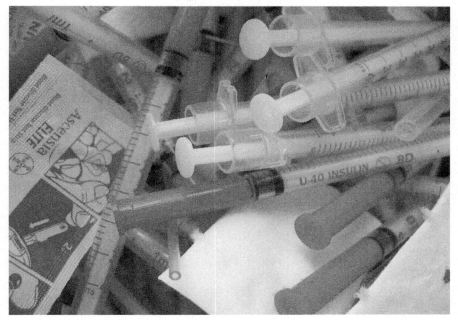

This chapter takes a look at some of the complementary and alternative medicines and treatments that may help people who are diagnosed with type II diabetes. You will also find some unconventional recommendations that may help prevent type II diabetes, or at least slow its progress. Just be reminded that no alternative treatments should be considered as a replacement for professional medical advice, and any drugs or pharmaceutical remedies must always be taken after proper consultation, examination, diagnosis and medical prescription by a licensed professional. It is also recommended that any alternative or complementary therapies must only be undertaken with the approval of your medical professional to make sure that all possible treatments being undertaken will not interact negatively with each other.

Reversing Type II Diabetes

Type 1 is something that can be managed but not necessarily reversed, type II however in many cases can be completely managed and controlled through dietary means. In this section, you will be given information on how to successfully reverse type II diabetes naturally.

Basically there are three food groups that you need to avoid and also a couple of food groups that you need to eat a lot of in order to do it. The great news is that it's going to be an enjoyable process; it will be very different than maybe what you've been recommended in the past. And according to many testimonies from diabetic people particularly diagnosed with type II is that reversing your condition just by tweaking your diet plans is effective, it works and can be done (IF you will it!)

There are technically four groups of food that would cause insulin resistance, and we're going to break that down in this section, but two of them fall under one larger sub-group. These are the following:

Food Groups that Causes Insulin Resistance and Leads You to Diabetes:

- Protein
- Saturated Fat
- Omega Six Fatty Acid
- Sugar

This might come as a surprise for many because the traditional "low – carb diet" that is recommended to diabetics is high in protein, however, it may not be as effective as you have been made to think. For you to understand the concept better and to prove how a natural and nutritious balance diet can reverse your type II diabetes, check out this experiment:

The Experiment

There was an experiment conducted around the 1920s wherein the researchers assigned four groups of people to four different diets; the first group was assigned to eat an all protein diet (consists of lean meat and egg whites), the second group was assigned to eat an all fat diet (made up of olive oil, butter, mayonnaise and cream), the third group was a fasted diet which was also called "starvation diet," where they eat nothing, and the last group was assigned to eat an all carbohydrate diet (consists of bread, potatoes, rice, bananas, oatmeal, candy or syrup).

The Results

After two days, the researchers tested the subjects with the glucose tolerance test. Please note that in this section, we will first discuss two of the largest subgroup of foods from the experiment that resulted to high levels of diabetes/insulin resistance:

All Protein Diet:

Fasted Blood Glucose (pre – protein diet test): 69

After 30 mins: 143 (qualified for diabetes; 140 is the threshold)

After 60 mins: 167

After 2 hours: 145

Conclusion: Protein alone can raise blood glucose and insulin levels

All Fat Diet:

Fasted Blood Glucose (pre – fat diet test): 83

After 30 mins: 170 (qualified for diabetes; 140 is the threshold)

After 60 mins: 206

After 2 hours: 173

Conclusion: Too much fat can cause profound insulin resistance at a very rapid rate. What the experiment found out is that if you frequently eat fatty foods, you can create diabetes in just 2 hours once the fat reaches your bloodstream. Among the four diet groups, the all fat diet group has the fastest and highest blood glucose reading.

What does it mean?

The reason that fat causes insulin resistance has to do with what has been dubbed as the "leaky membrane hypothesis. "All of our cells have a membrane, and that membrane needs to be kept fluid and flexible so that there can be an interchange of nutrients and other components such as glucose.

Most people know that saturated fats are solid at room temperature, what you may not know is that biochemically, saturated fats are fatty acids that are rigid in their structure which is what makes them solid at room temperature. And because of this, the saturated fat chain becomes aligned perpendicularly to the cell membrane and it blocks nutrients such as glucose from getting in and also makes the cell walls rigid. However, other fats such as omega 3 fatty acids have got several bonds in them that can make them change shapes very easily, so the omega fatty acids after being converted to DHA in the body can then combine itself into many different types of position.

The more double bonds that are inserted into a fat, the number of positions that it can get into drops off dramatically, this is why the omega 6 fatty acid (similar to saturated fats) such as those found in corn oil can also causes insulin resistance.

Ratio Matters

Even if you think that you are consuming high amounts of Omega 3 fatty acids, if you are still consuming high intakes of saturated fats and/or Omega 6 fatty acids that are often found in vegetable oil, olive oil, nuts, seeds, and avocados to name a few; those fats compete for the same enzymes that the Omega 3 fatty acids compete with. If you don't have proper ratios or amount of omega 3 intake, it will not convert properly.

Correct Ratio:

2.3 Omega 6/ Saturated Fat/Mono Fat is to 1 Omega 3 fatty acids

Make sure that you're not consuming more than 2.3 omega 6 fatty acids/saturated fats in the form of vegetable oil, seeds etc. If you are, then you have to decrease that dramatically and simultaneously increase your Omega 3 fatty acids intake in the form of flax seeds, chia seeds or other "plant fats." Fish oil is not recommended due to possible pollutants/mercury while fish is also not a good idea since protein can also increase your insulin resistance (refer to the results of the experiment above). Omega 3 found in plants fat or leafy greens can be converted to the DHA/EPA inside the body which can improve your condition dramatically.

According to many studies, doctors found out that vegans or vegetarians have sufficient levels of DHA/EPA in their bloodstream and tissues. It's not necessary to eat animal sources because it can contribute to the disease. Another factor that may prove omega 3 ineffective is triglycerides or excess fats; these fats are basically equivalent to vegetable oils. That's why even if you have proper intake of omega 3 fatty acids, and low intake of Omega 6, it may still not work because your own body is producing its own version of saturated fats! A combination of proper nutrition and weight loss is very crucial.

Healthy Carbohydrates

Based on the experiment, the group assigned to have an all carb diet has the lowest insulin resistance and didn't even reach the diabetes threshold. It also has the quickest sugar breakdown and has the most positive result compared to other food groups that was tested including the starvation group or those who didn't even take any food! The All – Carb diet has the best insulin sensitivity in all the groups. That's staggering! See the results below:

All Carb Diet:

Fasted Blood Glucose (pre – carb diet test): 84

After 30 mins: 118 (way below the 140 threshold)

After 60 mins: 113

After 2 hours: 96

Starvation/Fasting Diet:

Fasted Blood Glucose (pre – fasting diet test): 67

After 30 mins: 145 (qualified for diabetes; 140 threshold)

After 60 mins: 188

After 2 hours: 184

Based from the research, healthy carbohydrates such as sugar, brown rice, potatoes, oatmeal and fruit are not necessarily bad for diabetic people as what others claim. There is sucrose in these types of foods but it is minimal and does not contribute to triglycerides or is not converted to unnecessary fats, which is why the all – carb diet group in the research has the best glucose reading in the entire group.

Suggested Group of Foods To Reverse Type II Diabetes:

- Vegetables (green leafy veggies)
- Fruits
- Potatoes
- Rice (brown rice)
- Chia/ Flax Seeds

- Plant Fats

Suggested Group of Foods that Should Be Avoided

- Vegetable Oils
- Nuts and Seeds
- Saturated Fats in Coconut Oil and Animal Foods
- High Protein foods like Egg Whites and Lean Meats
- Sucrose in the form of table sugar
- Fructose found in Soft Drinks and Sweetened Beverages
- Highly Processed Foods

*It is highly recommended that you first consult with your physician about the particular foods (veggies/fruits etc.) that you need to eat to avoid conflict with your current condition or other possible underlying illnesses. The groups of foods listed here in this chapter are only suggestions and for educational purposes only. Other factors will be involved, make sure to plan your diet meal with your health care team.

In a nutshell, the only way you can reverse your type II diabetes or even prevent one before its onset is to eat the right amounts of foods particularly vegetables and fruits, keep tab on your blood sugar levels, stay away from fatty foods such as Omega 6/ saturated fat, exercise and stay fit to help your body absorb the right nutrients, follow your doctor's advice, and last but not least is none other than having the right attitude, strong mindset, and will power.

Reversing your type II diabetes according to most people will take a lot of discipline especially in the food you eat, and unwavering focus to reach your goal but once you do, the rewards are extremely gratifying. It will save you from financial ruin, improve your quality of life, and also take away that sense of doom for you and your family. Your burning desire to do all the necessary things will ultimately help you be free from diseases not just diabetes!

Chapter Seven: Future Treatments for Type II Diabetes

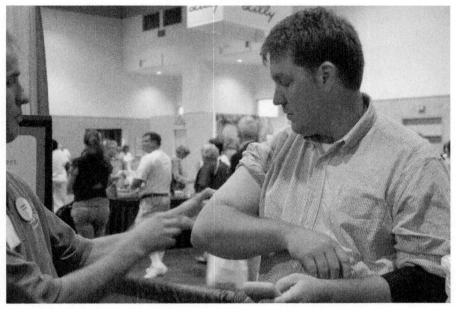

Researchers in the field of medicine had evolved in terms of knowledge and treatments in order to manage patients with type II diabetes. The advent of technology, and the educational advancement helped modern science propelled to staggering heights especially in terms of discoveries and various kinds of treatments; we've come a long way in just the past century if you think about it. However, the continuous development and research is still something every student of medicine – whether they are a medical practitioners, or general physicians as well as scientists – needs to do so that people diagnose with this condition can have various options (especially when it comes to long term treatments), more accurate knowledge than ever, and possibly inspire hope and the possibility of a permanent cure to those who were diagnosed with severe cases (diabetes with complications).

Type II diabetes usually appears to people who are obese or quite old (30 years and above), however it can already be detected at a very early age, and it can also be triggered at any stage of life. The most important thing is to recognized the tell – tale signs as early as you can so that you or your loved can be given treatment as soon as possible. The earlier the diagnosis, the earlier the treatments will be given, which in turn would be beneficial to the patients and to their families in the long run.

In this chapter, we will share with you the present challenges and struggles of health doctors on how to effectively treat the disease as well as what the future may hold for patients with diabetes in general – the possible technology – based treatments, new medical approaches, and how science can harness today's advanced technology in order to find a cure to the condition.

Current Challenges

According to many experts, like any other diseases, diabetes has its fair share of challenges. So before we focus on what the future may hold for diabetic patients, it's also essential to know the problems that physicians, medical professionals, scientists and even patients are facing today in terms of the current medical coverage and/or treatment. Knowing these things can help doctors and patients better understand the current status of the disease (not just on the physical aspect but also its economic sense) which can also eventually lead them to developing better ways in dealing with their patient's condition (physically/financially) and also possibly finding permanent cure in their patient's lifetime.

Challenge #1: Diabetes Medical Coverage and Supplies

According to Michelle Buysse, director of Commercial Care Management at Priority Health "patients not only need to pay for increasing insurance premiums but they also have to pay the additional cost of meeting deductibles, copays, and coinsurance."

What insurance companies are now doing for diabetic patients to overcome this challenge is to provide pricing transparency. Patients are now being given information about treatment options and its corresponding prices coupled with proper financial tools and support to have control over their healthcare.

Challenge #2: Medication Adherence

Experts and medical professionals learned that diabetic patients have difficulty in taking or adhering to the prescribed medication/treatment due to lack of awareness, financial cost, access and availability as well as competing priorities. Many experts suggest that the patients should work hand in hand with their health care team to address barriers and be able to come up with a plan that particularly works for the patients. They also added that patients should also at least attend diabetes seminars to get enough knowledge on how to properly deal with medications as well as self – management.

Challenge #3: Very Expensive Treatments

Just like any major illnesses, treating diabetes can lead a patient or its family to financial ruin or deplete most of its financial sources if not prevented or treated properly. The key is to detect the disease early so that early treatment options can be provided which could lessen and avoid further complications that could also lead to very expensive treatments. Diabetes is costly because it's the kind of disease that progresses and can affect vital bodily functions. The patient needs to change bad habits as soon as possible and again work with his/her medical "team."

Challenge #4: Pre-diabetics Currently Has No Disease Intervention

The American Diabetes Association reported that in the past 10 years, patients diagnosed with diabetes increased by about 40%. According to many medical experts, if there is no medical intervention, this percentage will definitely rise which could mean an unsustainable and unstable future for USA's healthcare system. CDC further reports that there are 30% of patients diagnosed with pre-diabetes that could progress to type II in the next three years.

What medical professionals and healthcare companies are now doing to at least reduce the risk of pre – diabetic patients progressing to type II is through partnering up with various health and local organizations to let these patients have access to the CDC's National Diabetes Prevention Program for free. This program consisting of lifestyle coaches, physicians, and medical practitioners aims to decrease the progression to as low as 58%. The program will tackle on how to properly educate patients in order for them to make the necessary lifestyle changes.

The Future Treatments for Diabetes

Artificial Pancreas

Just last year positive clinical trial results have come up for the artificial pancreas project. Artificial Pancreas is an embedded glucose sensor or an implantable glucose sensor coupled with an insulin pump, now there's a software algorithm that helps these two devices work together in the body but the end result is mostly passive, the only thing you have to do is to replace the battery every now and then and ensure that the device is full of insulin. If this works, it can be very helpful and transformative especially for those who have type 1 or type II diabetes.

Encapsulated Replacement Beta Cells

This procedure is essentially taking donor cells, putting them in a device and embedding it in the body wherein your immune system does not attack those cells. The goal is to normalize islet function. However, there could be limited donors for pancreatic islet cells but encapsulated beta cells may reduce immune response. It's more or less having a "different" pancreas.

Glucose Responsive Insulin

This technology can replace frequent insulin shots per day. Glucose responsive insulin aims for the patient to just have one dose or one shot of insulin that could last you through the day without having to carry around the needles or being constantly reminded to puncture yourself to measure your blood sugar and give yourself insulin shots.

The goals of researchers for this technology is that every time a diabetic person consumed a meal, and whenever the blood sugar rises as you wake up, the patient will be able to vary the dose depending on the body's need at any given time. Glucose responsive insulin may replace basal and mealtime insulin with just 1 daily injection. If it works it could be another breakthrough for diabetes.

Stem Cells

Stem cells involve the transformation of cells within your own body into cells that are capable of reproducing insulin when your blood sugar goes up. There have been various attempts in producing these technology or procedure through using embryonic cells, fetal cells and adult stem cells. Scientists have been testing all kinds of technologies in small mammals, using test tube procedures to make liver cells convert into insulin secreting cells. Lots of researchers and scientists are currently working on this innovation and in a few years you can expect to see various treatments involving living cells producing insulin for short – term or long – term use, it could be cells donated from a cell line, it could come from the patient's own body but most likely insulin will be produce in the body through using stem cells or technology similar to it.

Nanotechnology

Imagine putting one capsule into the body and have it take care of diabetes for you, no more pin pricks, and no more insulin injections. It just stays there for as long as that patient needs it. The pancreas does many things but its most important function is to regulate the levels of sugar in your body, and it does it through producing insulin.

What nanotechnology can potentially do is take the cells of the pancreas, the ones that secrete insulin, and scientists place them in a tiny capsule that is nano-porous, what that means is that the capsule have extremely tiny holes, and these holes allow for insulin that is released by the cells to come out into the body but it is small enough to keep out all the things that might attack those cells. The small device square capsule that scientists are currently developing has a central reservoir that can fit millions of cells and the back of the reservoir has tiny nanopores.

Researchers already have a prototype to help illustrate their point. The small rectangles in the prototype consist of millions of nanopores. According to researchers, these nanopores resembles a tea bag that you put in a hot water, the hot water then flows to the tea bag which releases the tea molecules that are contained in that netting. It's almost the same with the nano capsule but the difference is that there is (blood) sugar that comes into the capsule, and it alerts the cells inside to secrete insulin. According to these scientists, the real benefit of nanotechnology is creating small pores that can only allow insulin to go out but does not allow large immune cells or antibodies to come in.

Bonus Chapter:

Famous People Who Have Type Two Diabetes

Diabetes is a disease that can affect one's life negatively in the long run. It's a progressive condition that can also lead to other complications and fatality. However, for some people they learned how to manage and deal with this common illness and not let the disease stop them from living a great and purposeful life.

In this bonus chapter, you will get to know some of the most famous Hollywood celebrities who were diagnosed with type II diabetes, but still somehow were able to manage their condition, and live normal (and quite glamorous) lives. We'll give you a list of notable Hollywood celebs, artists, directors, musicians, inventors, politicians etc. that was previously diagnosed with the disease and/or managing their type II diabetes. You can get inspiration from them, and may also realize that you are not fighting alone; some of your favorite idols are also battling the same condition. Cheer up and don't let diabetes drag you down!

Notable Hollywood Celebrities diagnosed with Type II Diabetes:

1. Tom Hanks

History: Hanks revealed that he was recently diagnosed with type two during his interview with David Letterman.
Profession: Television director, Television producer, Film Producer, Screenwriter, Actor
Known For: Angles and Demons, The Da Vinci Code, Forrest Gump, Saving Private Ryan, The Green Mile

2. Halle Berry

History: Halle Berry was diagnosed with Type II diabetes at a young age. According to her, as soon as she found out she changed her diet drastically.
Profession: Television producer, Film Producer, Model, Actor, Voice acting
Known For: X-Men: The Last Stand, Cloud Atlas, X-Men 2, X-Men: Days of Future Past

3. Elvis Presley

History: When the rock star found out, he was actually shocked; unfortunately he didn't changed his lifestyle which is why many people think diabetes contributed to his early death.

Profession: Musician, Actor, Singer

Known For: Love Me Tender, Blue Hawaii, Jailhouse Rock, Viva Las Vegas

4. Larry King

History: The legend broadcaster stopped smoking and drastically changed his lifestyle after being diagnosed with type II diabetes.

Profession: Talk show host, Journalist, Radio personality, Actor, Voice acting

Known For: Larry King Now! CNN's Larry King Live

5. George Lucas

History: Lucas was diagnosed with a mild case of type II diabetes recently.

Profession: Television producer, Entrepreneur, Film Producer, Screenwriter, Cinematographer

Known For: Star Wars: Episode VI - Return of the Jedi, Indiana Jones and the Last Crusade, Star Wars: Episode II - Attack of the Clones, Star Wars: Episode IV - A New Hope

6. Drew Carey

History: Carey successfully reversed type II diabetes through living a healthy lifestyle.
Profession: Comedian, Television producer, Game Show Host, Screenwriter, Actor
Known For: The Price Is Right, Whose Line Is It Anyway? The Aristocrats

7. Thomas Edison

History: The famous inventor died in 1931 from complications of type II diabetes
Profession: Businessperson, Entrepreneur, Film Producer, Inventor, Scientist
Known For: Discovering electricity and the light bulb, has the most patented inventions in the world

8. Johnny Cash

History: Cash died at the age of 71 due to complications of type II diabetes.
Profession: Songwriter, Musician, Singer-songwriter, Author, Actor
Known For: Django Unchained, Walk the Line, Dawn of the Dead, Gone in Sixty Seconds

9. Mike Huckabee

History: Politician, Mike Huckabee, reportedly changed his diet to reverse his type II diabetes. He also regularly exercises to maintain his healthy lifestyle.
Profession: Public speaker, Commentator, Politician, Musician, Author
Known For: Huckabee, Fox and Friends, An Inconvenient Tax, Action Hero Makeover

10. Paula Deen

History: Famous Chef Paula Deen adapted a new diet to help treat her type II diabetes
Profession: Cook, TV chef, Restaurateur, Author, Actor
Known For: Paula's Best Dishes, Paula's Home Cooking, Paula Goes to Hollywood, Paula's Party

11. Sherry Shepherd

History: After being diagnosed with type II diabetes, talk show host Sherry Shepherd adapted a healthy lifestyle and also lost 40 pounds to help her treat the disease.
Profession: Comedian, Actor, Presenter, TV Personality

Known For: The View, Precious, Less than Perfect, Madagascar: Escape 2 Africa

12. Paul Sorvino

History: Actor, Paul Sorvino is continuously fighting the disease with the help of her daughter, Mira Sorvino.

Profession: Opera Singer, Sculptor, Activist, Copywriter, Television director

Known For: Goodfellas, Romeo + Juliet, Repo! The Genetic Opera, The Rocketeer

13. Randy Jackson

History: Since being diagnosed with type II diabetes, Jackson now spend his free time educating people about it.

Profession: Bassist, Record producer, Television producer, A&R executive, Musician

Known For: American Idol, America's Best Dance Crew, Soul Men, The Sing-Off, A Fairly Odd Movie: Grow Up

14. Mikhail Gorbachev

History: Russian leader was reportedly diagnosed with a severe case of type II diabetes and is still combatting the disease.

Profession: Politician, Lawyer

Known For: Faraway, So Close! Here to Stay, Svoboda po russki, The 11th Hour

15. H.G. Wells

History: Wells was a diabetic which led him to founding Diabetes UK.

Profession: Journalist, Historian, Novelist, Writer, Teacher

Known For: War of the World, The Time Machine, Things to Come

Index

H

I

L

S

T

V

Photo References

Page Photo by user Practical Cures via Flickr.com, https://www.flickr.com/photos/practicalcures/24298761582/

Page Photo by user Practical Cures via Flickr.com, https://www.flickr.com/photos/practicalcures/24111411340/in/photostream/

Page Photo by user Jaytaix via Pixabay.com, https://pixabay.com/en/nurse-diabetes-diabetic-test-a1c-527615/

Page Photo by user Alan Levine via Flickr.com, https://www.flickr.com/photos/cogdog/32672740093/

Page Photo by user stevepb via Pixabay.com, https://pixabay.com/en/diabetes-blood-sugar-diabetic-528678/

Page Photo by user via Lindsay Attaway Flickr.com, https://www.flickr.com/photos/lindsayloveshermac/7641036682/

Page Photo by user Geralt via Pixabay.com, https://pixabay.com/en/insulin-insulin-syringe-syringe-113200/

Page Photo by user Diabetes Education Events via Flickr.com, https://www.flickr.com/photos/tcoyd/5009449523/

References

5 Future Treatments for Type II Diabetes –
Type II Diabetes.com
https://type2diabetes.com/living/5-future-treatments-type-2-diabetes/

A complete of List of Diabetes Medications –
Healthline.com
http://www.healthline.com/health/diabetes/medications-list#overview1

Diabetes – NHS UK
http://www.nhs.uk/Conditions/Diabetes/Pages/Diabetes.aspx

Diabetes – MedlinePlus.gov
https://medlineplus.gov/diabetes.html

Diabetic Emergencies – Emergency Care for You
http://www.emergencycareforyou.org/Emergency-101/Emergencies-A-Z/Diabetic-Emergencies/

Diabetes Milletus – Wikipedia.org

https://en.wikipedia.org/wiki/Diabetes_mellitus

Diabetes Milletus Type II – Wikipedia.org
https://en.wikipedia.org/wiki/Diabetes_mellitus_type_2

Diabetes Overview – Webmd.com
http://www.webmd.com/diabetes/

Diabetes Treatment History Timeline – World History
    Project.org
https://worldhistoryproject.org/topics/diabetes-treatment-
    history

Diabetes: Symptoms, Causes and Treatments –
Medical News Today
http://www.medicalnewstoday.com/info/diabetes

How to Reverse Diabetes Naturally in 30 days or less –
    Dr. Axe.com
https://draxe.com/how-to-reverse-diabetes-naturally-in-30-
    days-or-less/

Natural Progression of Type II Diabetes – Diabetes
    Digest.com

http://diabetesdigest.com/living-with-type-2-diabetes-progression/

Natural Remedies for Type II Diabetes – Webmd.com
http://www.webmd.com/diabetes/type-2-diabetes-guide/natural-remedies-type-2-diabetes#1

Reversing Type II Diabetes With Natural Therapies – Today's Dietitian
http://www.todaysdietitian.com/newarchives/111412p28.shtml

Timeline 1900 – 1950 – Diapedia.org
https://www.diapedia.org/introduction-to-diabetes-mellitus/1104709121/timeline-1900-1950

Type II Diabetes – MedlinePlus.gov
https://medlineplus.gov/ency/article/000313.htm

Type II Diabetes Overview – Mayoclinic.org
http://www.mayoclinic.org/diseases-conditions/type-2-diabetes/home/ovc-20169860

Type II Diabetes Progression – Diabetes Forecast Organization

http://www.diabetesforecast.org/2015/sep-oct/type-2-
  diabetes-progression.html

Type II Diabetes: The Basics – Webmd.com
http://www.webmd.com/diabetes/type-2-diabetes-
  guide/type-2-diabetes

Understanding Type II Diabetes – Healthline.com
http://www.healthline.com/health/type-2-diabetes

What is Diabetes – Diabetes Researh Organization
https://www.diabetesresearch.org/what-is-diabetes

What Kind of Type II Diabetes Do You Have? – Diabetes
  Self – Management.com
https://www.diabetesselfmanagement.com/blog/kind-type-
  2-diabetes/

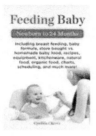

Feeding Baby
Cynthia Cherry
978-1941070000

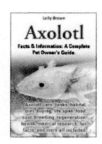

Axolotl
Lolly Brown
978-0989658430

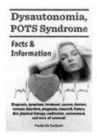

Dysautonomia, POTS
Syndrome
Frederick Earlstein
978-0989658485

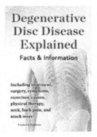

Degenerative Disc
Disease Explained
Frederick Earlstein
978-0989658485

Sinusitis, Hay Fever,
Allergic Rhinitis Explained
Frederick Earlstein
978-1941070024

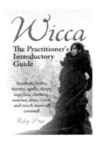

Wicca
Riley Star
978-1941070130

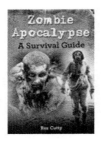

Zombie Apocalypse
Rex Cutty
978-1941070154

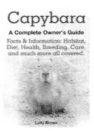

Capybara
Lolly Brown
978-1941070062

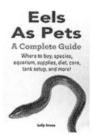

Eels As Pets
Lolly Brown
978-1941070167

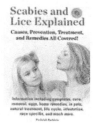

Scabies and Lice Explained
Frederick Earlstein
978-1941070017

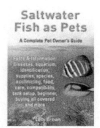

Saltwater Fish As Pets
Lolly Brown
978-0989658461

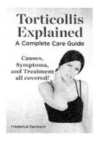

Torticollis Explained
Frederick Earlstein
978-1941070055

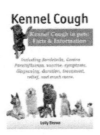

Kennel Cough
Lolly Brown
978-0989658409

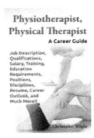

Physiotherapist, Physical
Therapist
Christopher Wright
978-0989658492

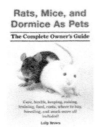

Rats, Mice, and Dormice
As Pets
Lolly Brown
978-1941070079

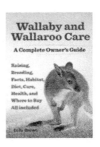

Wallaby and Wallaroo Care
Lolly Brown
978-1941070031

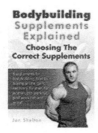

Bodybuilding Supplements
Explained
Jon Shelton
978-1941070239

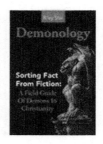

Demonology
Riley Star
978-19401070314

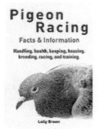

Pigeon Racing
Lolly Brown
978-1941070307

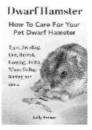

Dwarf Hamster
Lolly Brown
978-1941070390

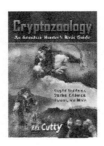

Cryptozoology
Rex Cutty
978-1941070406

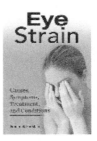

Eye Strain
Frederick Earlstein
978-1941070369

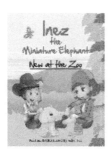

Inez The Miniature Elephant
Asher Ray
978-1941070353

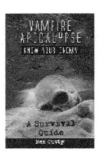

Vampire Apocalypse
Rex Cutty
978-1941070321